# Cambridge Elements

Elements of Improving Quality and Safety in Healthcare
edited by
Mary Dixon-Woods,[*] Katrina Brown,[*] Sonja Marjanovic,[†]
Tom Ling,[†] Ellen Perry,[*] and Graham Martin[*]
*THIS Institute (The Healthcare Improvement Studies Institute)
†RAND Europe

# COLLABORATION-BASED APPROACHES

## Graham Martin and Mary Dixon-Woods

THIS Institute (The Healthcare Improvement Studies Institute),
University of Cambridge

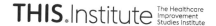

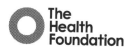

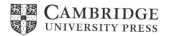

# CAMBRIDGE
## UNIVERSITY PRESS

University Printing House, Cambridge CB2 8BS, United Kingdom

One Liberty Plaza, 20th Floor, New York, NY 10006, USA

477 Williamstown Road, Port Melbourne, VIC 3207, Australia

314–321, 3rd Floor, Plot 3, Splendor Forum, Jasola District Centre, New Delhi – 110025, India

103 Penang Road, #05–06/07, Visioncrest Commercial, Singapore 238467

Cambridge University Press is part of the University of Cambridge.

It furthers the University's mission by disseminating knowledge in the pursuit of education, learning, and research at the highest international levels of excellence.

www.cambridge.org
Information on this title: www.cambridge.org/9781009236829
DOI: 10.1017/9781009236867

© THIS Institute 2022

First published 2022

*A catalogue record for this publication is available from the British Library.*

ISBN 978-1-009-23682-9 Paperback
ISSN 2754-2912 (online)
ISSN 2754-2904 (print)

Cambridge University Press has no responsibility for the persistence or accuracy of URLs for external or third-party internet websites referred to in this publication and does not guarantee that any content on such websites is, or will remain, accurate or appropriate.

Every effort has been made in preparing this Element to provide accurate and up-to-date information that is in accord with accepted standards and practice at the time of publication. Although case histories are drawn from actual cases, every effort has been made to disguise the identities of the individuals involved. Nevertheless, the authors, editors, and publishers can make no warranties that the information contained herein is totally free from error, not least because clinical standards are constantly changing through research and regulation. The authors, editors, and publishers therefore disclaim all liability for direct or consequential damages resulting from the use of material contained in this Element. Readers are strongly advised to pay careful attention to information provided by the manufacturer of any drugs or equipment that they plan to use.

# Collaboration-Based Approaches

## Elements of Improving Quality and Safety in Healthcare

DOI: 10.1017/9781009236867
First published online: August 2022

Graham Martin and Mary Dixon-Woods
*THIS Institute (The Healthcare Improvement Studies Institute),
University of Cambridge*
**Author for correspondence:** Graham Martin,
graham.martin@thisinstitute.cam.ac.uk

**Abstract:** Collaboration-based approaches to healthcare improvement attract much attention. They involve networks of people coming together to cooperate around a common interest, with shared goals of improving care and mutual learning. Long-standing examples of collaborative approaches have been associated with some success in improving outcomes and reducing harm. The evidence for their effectiveness and cost-effectiveness, however, remains inconsistent and contingent on the circumstances in which they are deployed and how they are used for what purpose. Several models for collaboration have been developed, varying in structure, format, and balance between internal leadership and external control. This Element focuses on two approaches: quality improvement collaboratives and communities of practice. The authors explore evidence of their impact on health outcomes, and evidence about how best to organise and implement collaboration-based approaches. Using examples of more and less successful collaborations, this Element offers guidance on the key challenges involved in using collaboration-based approaches to improve healthcare. This title is also available as Open Access on Cambridge Core.

**Keywords:** collaboration, quality improvement collaboratives, clinical networks, communities of practice, clinical communities

ISBNs: 9781009236829 (PB), 9781009236867 (OC)
ISSNs: 2754-2912 (online), 2754-2904 (print)

# Contents

# 1 Introduction

In this Element, we identify the potential and challenges of using collaboration-based approaches to support improvement in healthcare. We review a range of approaches, summarising some of the evidence about their role, value, and limitations. We conclude by discussing the implications for those considering using such approaches in practice. Our focus is on collaboration-based approaches led primarily by healthcare staff, since this is where much of the academic literature has focused. Some other approaches focus on the contribution of patients and carers – for example, those addressed in the Element on co-producing and co-designing.[1]

# 2 What Are Collaboration-Based Approaches?

One of the most enduring lessons of research in healthcare improvement is that improving quality requires systems for sharing knowledge, coordinating and organising activity, and encouraging cultures that are supportive of improvement. In this context, the promise of collaboration-based approaches to improvement has become a focus of increasing interest, activity, and study.[2]

Though the literature on collaboration is rapidly growing and developing, a universal definition has proven elusive. In part, this is because, as we shall see, many different collaborative forms have emerged. The unifying feature of collaboration-based approaches however is that they involve groups working together around shared improvement goals.

Another crucial feature of these approaches is that they are based on networks.[3,4] Networks are ubiquitous in everyday life – they connect parents whose children attend the same school, colleagues who share the same professional background or workplace, and people who play a team sport, for instance. Networks enable multiple forms of relationship-based exchange, allowing people, for example, to share contacts or exchange favours.[2] They have a particularly important role in the speedy and efficient exchange of knowledge,[4] including the know-how formed within a particular community. This kind of 'non-canonical'[5] knowledge (the sort that concerns how things are really done in practice) is especially valuable because it is frequently implicit or unspoken, practice-based, and often difficult to articulate or formally describe.[6] Networks are not, of course, just circuits for information exchange.[7,8] They also exert powerful effects on norms, values, and behaviour – in other words, the culture of the group involved.[9]

Though a collaboration cannot exist without a network, a network on its own does not equate to a collaboration. Networks may exist without any common mission, but collaborations are purposeful. Additional characteristics of collaborations in healthcare contexts include a commitment to cooperating and contributing in pursuit of that purpose and an ethos of learning. These features tend to foster trust and reciprocity: if a collaboration works well, it can generate a virtuous circle in which mutual benefits encourage further investment of time and effort, resulting in further benefits. We therefore offer the following definition.

> *In healthcare, a collaboration-based approach to improvement involves a network of people who come together to cooperate around a common interest, with a shared goal of improving care and mutual learning.*

In this basic formulation, collaboration-based approaches can be readily recognised as consistent with the long-standing principles and values of community that underpin the healthcare professions,[10] particularly when they are empowered to set their own rules and enforce them through peer influence.[11,12]

Several types of collaboration-based approach to healthcare improvement can be identified, ranging from informal communities of practice at one end of the spectrum through to managed clinical networks at the other, with many other forms (e.g. quality improvement collaboratives, clinical communities) somewhere in the middle. They vary in their origins, degree of formality, and exclusivity of membership, and in the methods used to achieve their goals. Although collaborations are sometimes described as professionally led[13] or bottom-up[14] improvement approaches, the degree to which they exhibit these features varies. In Section 3, we explore a small selection of the various approaches available.

## 3 A Selection of Collaboration-Based Approaches

Collaboration-based approaches to healthcare improvement vary in form and origin. Some were developed primarily in a healthcare context; others have their roots in quite different fields. They also vary in the extent to which they are focused explicitly and primarily on improving quality and patient safety, the extent to which they are naturally occurring or deliberately formed, and the formality with which they are organised and coordinated.

To illustrate this range, we describe four collaboration-based approaches: quality improvement collaboratives, managed clinical networks, communities of practice, and clinical communities. These approaches are not exhaustive. They are chosen because they vary in how much they tend towards control, self-organisation, and professional ownership.

### 3.1 Quality Improvement Collaboratives

Some collaboration-based approaches are highly organised, featuring an extensive and well-documented infrastructure, prescriptions for organisation, and specified activities, events for interaction, and timetables. Among the most prominent and best-known examples of this kind of approach are quality improvement collaboratives.

Collaboratives typically focus on a specific clinical topic (such as a presenting condition, pathway, or intervention) – often one in which large variations in care or gaps between current and best practice are known to exist. They involve creating a network of people from several organisations (or occasionally within organisations) and multi-professional teams around defined improvement goals. A core group or faculty works on periodically convening members of the network, coordinating its members, establishing shared goals, and providing infrastructural support, such as a database or registry to which participants submit data, using indicators with standardised definitions and methodologies.[15,16] Participating sites receive feedback, usually benchmarked against other sites, and attend face-to-face or virtual meetings to discuss progress and identify interventions that might be used to support improvement. These features, while typical, are not invariable: quality improvement collaboratives take many different forms.

### 3.1.1 Growth of Collaboratives in North America

Some of the early collaboratives originated in North America.[15] An important example is the Vermont Oxford Network.[17] This not-for-profit organisation was established in the late 1980s to improve the quality and safety of care for newborn infants and families through a coordinated programme of research, education, and quality improvement. Now involving more than 1,200 hospitals worldwide (including around 800 in the USA), it is organised around a network of healthcare professionals who work together as an interdisciplinary community. All members of the network contribute data to high-quality databases on interventions and outcomes for infants under their care. Key to the approach is the use of uniform and standardised definitions for data collection. Members are given detailed, confidential, risk-adjusted reports that allow them to track their data over time and measure the performance of their unit against others.

The Vermont Oxford Network has much in common with another well-known collaborative: the Northern New England Cardiovascular Disease Study Group, also founded in the late 1980s. A voluntary consortium, it initially focused on hospitals across three US states that were seeking to improve outcomes of coronary artery bypass graft surgery. By gathering standardised data from all hospitals, the collaborative identified variations in mortality after surgery that could not be explained by case-mix. It undertook a three-component improvement programme, which involved giving benchmarked performance feedback to participating centres, training courses in continuous quality improvement, and team-based visits to all sites.[18]

A similar, though somewhat later, movement took place in the US state of Michigan in 1997. Hospitals began to work with Blue Cross Blue Shield of Michigan (a health insurer), which owns the Blue Care Network (a health maintenance organisation), to study variation in outcomes of angioplasty services. By 2004, Blue Cross Blue Shield of Michigan was investing in statewide quality improvement initiatives in a variety of clinical specialties. The Michigan collaboratives are now a large-scale enterprise, involving programmes across several different clinical fields (Box 1). All the programmes use clinical registries, with hospitals and clinicians submitting data and receiving feedback on their performance from their registry coordinating centre. Participating healthcare organisations convene to interpret and review their data, often focusing on variations. Best practices are identified and implemented across regions.[19]

Several of these kinds of large, often statewide collaborative have endured over time, with many – perhaps crucially – distinguished by their commitment

---

**BOX 1 THE MICHIGAN COLLABORATIVES' PROGRAMMES**

The Michigan collaboratives' programmes have reported some striking improvements in the quality and safety of healthcare services, sometimes outperforming both secular trends and improvements made by other improvement programmes. One example is the Michigan Surgical Quality Collaborative. Focusing on general and vascular surgery, it is the largest and most mature of the Michigan collaboratives. Between 2005 and 2009, participating hospitals reduced risk-adjusted morbidity rates (the primary outcome measure of the American College of Surgeons' National Surgical Quality Improvement Program, NSQIP) from 13.1% to 10.5%, outperforming results achieved by participants in NSQIP.[19]

The Michigan Bariatric Surgery Collaborative has also produced impressive improvements, including a reduction in the overall rate of perioperative complications among participating hospitals from 8.7% to 6.6% in the first two years of the programme (2007–09).[19] More recently, in 2012–14, the Michigan Urological Surgery Improvement Collaborative achieved a 53% reduction in infection-related hospital admissions following transrectal prostate biopsy, among participating hospitals.[20]

Key to these collaboratives' achievements seems to be the use of high-quality, clinically relevant data; site visits; collaborative learning; treating practice variation between hospitals as natural experiments in what works and what doesn't; rapid and robust assessments of relationships between process changes and outcomes; and improvements in safety culture associated with peer-norming effects.[19]

to research as well as to quality improvement. The Vermont Oxford Network, now over 30 years in existence, continues to meet three times a year. As well as supporting quality improvement, it uses its platform to conduct observational studies, intervention studies, and research on the role of differences in the structure and organisation of units in explaining patient outcomes.[21] By so doing, it has made a substantial contribution to the evidence base for neonatal care. The Northern New England Cardiovascular Disease Study Group remains similarly active. The Michigan collaboratives' programmes, though newer, continue to thrive, with large numbers of published studies.

A rather different, though very popular, model of a collaborative is the more time-limited, topic-specific approach offered by the Institute for Healthcare Improvement's (IHI) Breakthrough Series. Conceived by the IHI's founders in 1994, a Breakthrough Series collaborative is time-bound (often in the range of 6–15 months) and usually involves three face-to-face learning sessions between participants drawn from several organisations. Central to the theory of change – the assumptions about how its activities will give rise to the intended outcomes (see the Element on evaluation[22]) – is that those involved must have a clear objective, a clear means of measuring whether that objective has been achieved, and a notion of what is needed to make that change happen. Box 2 summarises the blueprint for running a Breakthrough Series collaborative.[24] The detailed blueprint includes recommendations about the numbers of organisations and individuals that should be involved, the timing of meetings, the relationship to other improvement methods (such as the IHI's Model for Improvement), the role of expert faculty in guiding improvement, and the intended outputs and outcomes.[24] Various how-to guides are available.[25,26]

---

BOX 2 KEY ELEMENTS OF THE IHI'S BREAKTHROUGH SERIES COLLABORATIVE APPROACH

(1) **Topic selection:** the topic should be ripe for improvement efforts: for example, there may be a demonstrable gap between evidence and its use in practice that has important consequences for patients and that is tractable to improvement.

(2) **Faculty:** as part of the package of support available to organisations, 5–15 experts in relevant disciplines, including those with improvement expertise, are asked by the collaborative's convenors to form a faculty of subject matter experts and individual clinicians. The faculty develops content for the collaborative – for example, aims, measurement strategies, and the evidence-based changes to be implemented.

(3) **Enrolment of participating organisations and teams:** organisations are asked to identify multidisciplinary teams to join the collaborative. Senior leaders in organisations are expected to provide guidance and encouragement and to take responsibility for sustaining improvement after the collaborative dissolves. Participating teams are expected to attend collaborative meetings and activities, seek to implement changes in their own practices, and promote changes as standard practice locally.

(4) **Learning sessions and action periods:** a typical collaborative involves three face-to-face meetings between participating teams and expert faculty. These are interspersed with action periods, when teams seek to test and implement changes and collect data on their impact. The first learning session presents a vision for improvement and outlines the specific changes needed to achieve it. During the second and third learning sessions, teams report on their successes and failures and learn from each other to improve their future efforts (e.g. through plenary sessions, workshops, and informal dialogue and exchange).

(5) **Quality improvement methods:** the IHI recommends that collaboratives use the Model for Improvement (see the Element on the IHI approach[23]) during action periods to ensure a systematic approach to change. This involves agreeing on specific and measurable aims, collecting data and measuring improvement over time, identifying key changes that are expected to result in improvement, running a series of plan-do-study-act cycles that seek to test the changes and their results, and learning from the findings to inform further efforts.

(6) **Summative outputs:** at the end of the collaborative, teams have a final face-to-face meeting to present their results to each other and to groups beyond the participating organisations, ensuring wide dissemination of learning and spread of ideas.

(7) **Measurement and evaluation:** throughout the process, participating teams are expected to maintain run charts tracking their progress through time, and faculty members review monthly reports from participating teams to keep track of the collaborative's overall progress.

Adapted from the IHI.[24]

As we discuss later, studies of Breakthrough Series collaboratives provide useful insights into whether and how they work. However, Breakthrough Series collaboratives do not themselves, unlike some of the collaboratives mentioned earlier, set out with research as one of their primary goals. Their outputs are usually (though not invariably) published as quality improvement reports[27] rather than as research articles.

### 3.1.2 Collaborative Approaches in the UK

The UK has not had the same trajectory as the USA in terms of adopting and using collaboration-based approaches. Although Breakthrough Series collaboratives were the government's chosen strategy for improvement in the National Health Service (NHS) in the early 2000s and were promoted by the NHS Modernisation Agency, they struggled to be adopted at scale. Those that were initiated tended to suffer from various problems, including haphazard reporting of outcomes and poor collection and interpretation of data.[28] Some important examples of collaboratives nonetheless emerged from this period, including the Cancer Services Collaborative and the Orthopaedic Services Collaborative, but while they did valuable work, neither may have delivered fully on the promise of the approach.[28]

Perhaps the UK's nearest equivalents to the large US statewide collaboratives led by clinicians (such as the Michigan collaboratives' programmes) are the audits and registries established by royal colleges, professional societies, and others from the late twentieth century onwards. An early example is the monitoring of survival rates after cardiac surgery through voluntary submission of data to the Society of Cardiothoracic Surgery, which began in 1977.[29] Clinical audit in the UK, as in many countries, is now a large-scale enterprise involving around 70 national exercises in collecting process and outcome data across a range of settings with many stakeholders. Around 30 are operated by professional groupings (such as the royal colleges) as part of a national managed scheme: the National Clinical Audit and Patient Outcomes Programme. Funded by NHS England and the Welsh Government, these audits are commissioned by the Healthcare Quality Improvement Partnership, a consortium comprising the Academy of Medical Royal Colleges, the Royal College of Nursing, and National Voices (a patients' charity).

Originally, the early registries and audits in the UK were largely voluntary, professionally led enterprises. Participation in the National Clinical Audit and Patient Outcomes Programme is now mandatory for NHS organisations in England, following the introduction of a contractual requirement in 2012. Data from the audits can be mobilised for several purposes, including quality assurance, pay-for-performance schemes, and inspection and regulation. As a result, these audits have assumed a somewhat hybrid character: though many are still led and organised by professional groups, they are funded by government and have become part of the NHS system of performance management. Though many audits have demonstrated improvement in processes and outcomes over time, they have, particularly as they have been absorbed into the performance-management architecture, lost some of the features of collaboration that characterised the early efforts. Further, the principal means of quality improvement has often remained data collection and feedback (see the Element on audit, feedback, and behaviour change[30]), and the deployment of structured quality improvement methods and collaboration-based efforts remains patchy and inconsistent.

Some important collaboration-based examples with features similar to those of long-term collaboratives, like the Michigan collaboratives' programmes, have nonetheless emerged. They include the National Audit Projects run by the Royal College of Anaesthetists, which have addressed important problems in surgery using a characteristically community-based approach that includes clinicians and patients as part of the collaboration.[31]

## 3.2 Managed Clinical Networks

Some collaboration-based approaches to improvement have been in some sense *managed* from the start: rather than originating from voluntary association between individuals or professional groups with a common interest or goal, they have been initiated by policymakers or managers.

In the UK, the Labour government of 1997–2010 is particularly associated with a renewed interest in the power of collaboration. Key thinkers had become disillusioned with the effects of both traditional hierarchical approaches to governing public services and the market-based, competition-oriented reforms that had been introduced from the late 1980s onwards.[32] Collaboration-based approaches were seen as drawing on professionals' intrinsic motivation to provide high-quality services and to work together to improve provision. The creation of networks between organisations and professionals was also seen as a key way of ensuring that public services could address 'wicked issues': challenges that are complex and multifaceted, and are therefore beyond the ability of any one organisation to handle in isolation.

These collaborative networks were introduced in various fields to facilitate joint effort and knowledge sharing, with the aim of solving problems and improving public services.[33] A prominent example in healthcare is the introduction of managed clinical networks in cancer provision and other areas of the

NHS in the early 2000s, to promote 'interorganizational collaboration, partnerships and a weakening of the vertical lines' of accountability.[34] Cancer networks were introduced in response to policy reports that high-quality care was being impeded by poor dissemination of evidence and good practice. The networks sought to formalise and provide an infrastructure for lateral relationships that had previously been informal and patchy, creating opportunities for dialogue among staff and organisations that might promote knowledge sharing, and facilitating peer review to inform service improvements. They aimed to go beyond building links between clinicians separated by organisational boundaries and to provide a basis for agreements about responsibilities, care pathways, and service specifications.[35]

The cancer networks were better resourced financially and managerially than many forms of collaboration. But the available evidence suggests that their impact was limited by the wider context in which they were introduced, and by the form in which they were realised. For example, Addicott et al. report that, for all their collaborative intent, cancer networks were infused with the performance management culture that was dominant at the time.[34] Though originally conceived as a vehicle for professional education and multidisciplinary training and development, their focus quickly shifted towards coordination of services and the measurement of performance.[36] The result was that the networks became, in many cases, little more than an extra vehicle for the achievement of targets. Managerially controlled rather than professionally owned, they were criticised for 'the managerial element driving out some of the pre-existing networks between clinicians'.[34]

An important lesson of managed clinical networks, therefore, is that the values and behaviours of a collaborative network can become dominated – perhaps even undermined – by hierarchical command, market-based competition, and other forms of directive control in the wider environment. As we discuss later, other collaboration-based approaches may face similar challenges.

## 3.3 Communities of Practice

If managed clinical networks are at one end of the spectrum of collaboration-based approaches, communities of practice are at the other. Developed in the field of educational psychology, the origins of the concept are distinctive. Lave and Wenger proposed the community of practice not as a planned way of making change, but as an analytical description of the way newcomers are socialised into different forms of community.[37]

These communities may be very different, including, for example, occupational groups (e.g. midwives) or people with a common interest or identity (e.g. Alcoholics Anonymous). What such groups have in common, argue Lave and Wenger, is that becoming a member involves a form of apprenticeship (which they term 'legitimate peripheral participation'), through which newcomers learn how to behave as well as what to do, and start to acquire a group identity,[37] primarily through informal learning and interaction. Communities of practice as first conceptualised, then, were not interventions (for improvement or any other purpose), and they were not developed in the context of healthcare. Lave and Wenger's contribution was to describe a process that took place naturally across several different kinds of settings.

Others quickly saw the relevance of the concept to other activities, including Brown and Duguid's famous reanalysis of a series of ethnographic studies of Xerox engineers.[5] This work characterised the knowledge-sharing activities of a group whose professional expertise was seemingly threatened by increasingly intelligent photocopiers (which could supposedly identify and fix faults themselves) and by increasingly copious instruction manuals. Brown and Duguid found that, far from becoming a simple matter of following instructions, the work of the engineer remained one where know-how was crucial – and where the community of colleagues, who shared lunch, phoned each other, or gathered for after-work drinks, was an essential resource. Collective knowledge shared with colleagues, including tacit knowledge (such as heuristics, top tips, and workarounds) was at least as important as explicit, formal information.

Several authors – including Wenger himself – have since developed the concept of the community of practice as a more intentional intervention, not just a naturally occurring phenomenon. While Wenger et al. maintain that communities of practice cannot be engineered by organisations, they can be cultivated: organisations can generate the conditions in which communities of practice can emerge and flourish, and create innovative work-related insights that benefit staff and organisations alike.[38]

Consequently, communities of practice represent a rather more open-ended approach to improvement than most other collaborative forms, as illustrated by the example in Box 3. They do not follow detailed instructions for how to organise and run themselves (in contrast to, for example, the Breakthrough Series approach). Communities of practice generally determine for themselves what they do, rather than having their activities chosen or imposed externally. Their interest is in developing sets of practices and capabilities, and they select areas of focus themselves on the basis of their work, knowledge, and commitment to the group.[41]

These are not hard-and-fast features. The labels in this field are often applied variably – for instance, we classified the Vermont Oxford Network as a quality

BOX 3 A COMMUNITY OF PRACTICE IN HEALTHCARE

Kilbride et al.[39] discuss the development of a community of practice during the redesign of a stroke service in London. Complementing project management and implementation, and allowing knowledge sharing and a network of relationships to emerge, the community of practice was seen as fundamental to the successful introduction of a new stroke unit. It demonstrated four important features:

- building an interprofessional stroke team (and breaching professional boundaries that had previously been rather impermeable)
- developing practice-based knowledge and skills in stroke care (particularly tacit knowledge about the *craft* of care – things that cannot readily be codified, as Brown and Duguid[5] emphasise)
- valuing the central role of the nurse in stroke care (particularly making visible the extent to which high-quality stroke care is dependent on the contribution of this role)
- creating an organisational climate for supporting improvement.

The community of practice came about not as a deliberate intervention, but rather emerged during the change process, facilitated by several features of how the change was organised. Team meetings 'often had no pre-arranged agenda but were problem focussed', offering a theme (or a 'practice' in Wenger-Trayner and Wenger-Trayner's[40] terms) around which the community could congregate.

Though it was difficult to attract people to take time out of busy schedules to attend such unstructured meetings at first, quick wins encouraged a range of colleagues to attend. The approach also fostered a sense of community: mutual commitment and a 'meaningful sense of shared identity that tied people beyond specific workplace exchanges'. Care was taken to nurture collegial relationships and to include the range of people affected by the changes, including managerial and clinical staff. Together, members of the community took the chance to think through the organisational implications of the change: what new competencies would be needed, what demands it would place on existing staff members, and how their coordination might need to change. The community of practice also fed back into the formal organisation of the change initiative, leading, for example, to the introduction of an interprofessional stroke committee comprising senior managers and stroke unit clinicians. This offered a means by which the community could influence wider organisational strategy.

Consistent with the original theory, the community of practice here was not the result of a formal decision or even intentional action: rather, it was 'fundamentally self-established, being composed of staff who originally worked in a dispersed service'. But in bridging professional boundaries and creating a sense of common purpose and mutual commitment, it ensured that social dynamics – which can so often derail change projects that look good on paper – supported a smooth redesign of the service.

improvement collaborative earlier, but it also self-identifies as a community of practice.[21] Moreover, as we see later in Section 5, some argue that the concept and language of communities of practice have increasingly been co-opted as a rather crude tool for knowledge management.

## 3.4 Clinical Communities

An evolution of collaboration-based approaches from the 2010s builds on learning about both the successes and limitations of quality improvement collaboratives, communities of practice, and network-based approaches more broadly: the clinical community approach (Box 4).[2] The clinical community attempts to find the right balance between the self-organising, member-led ethos that underlies the idea of collaboration, and the need for administrative and managerial support to help a collaboration achieve its objectives.[43] Box 5 presents an example of the approach in action, and what is needed to make it work.

---

BOX 4 PRINCIPLES OF CLINICAL COMMUNITIES

Aveling et al.[2] set out eight lessons for those seeking to develop clinical communities as a form of collaboration-based healthcare improvement.

(1) Foster a strong 'vertically integrating core': a coordinating group to organise the collaboration and keep it on course towards its objectives. Collaborations do not organise themselves, and leadership is crucial (to ensure both effective administration and, when needed, managerial clout – see point 7).

(2) Start from a clear theory of change, but be prepared to learn and modify. It is important to consider in advance how the clinical community is going to make change happen, but not everything can be anticipated.

(3) Identify and provide the right resources and training. Technical knowledge, tacit know-how (as emphasised in communities of practice), and skills in change management and leadership are key.

(4) Hold the community together, and recognise and deal with conflict and marginalisation. In practice, even highly functional communities tend to be 'fragmented, hierarchical and involve relationships of conflict': managing these tensions effectively is crucial to longevity and success.

(5) Foster a sense of community. Active intervention is required to identify a common goal and to develop relationships of mutual obligation.

(6) Collect and use data wisely. Good-quality data, and knowledge of how to make use of it, is vital to any improvement initiative (see also the Element on measurement for improvement[42]). Data show what needs to be done and help people to monitor their progress – and can provide the basis for healthy comparison across settings.

(7) Find the balance between hard and soft tactics. Persuasion, negotiation, and compromise are fundamental to collaboration-based approaches, but sometimes *harder* tactics are needed. Sometimes communities need protection from external performance pressures; at other times, they can be mobilised to reinforce the importance of improvement.

(8) Recognise the importance of context: local contexts can influence the likelihood of success and create supportive conditions. The wider context, such as organisational culture or national policy, is likely to influence the preoccupations and priorities of members.

BOX 5 CLINICAL COMMUNITIES IN ACTION

Aveling et al. compared two contrasting examples of clinical communities, deriving lessons about what is needed to make the approach work in practice.[43] Three areas of activity seem important in creating enduring communities with the capacity to achieve improvement.

• **Mobilising diverse groups:** both communities were successful in mobilising diverse groups of individuals from different backgrounds, including clinicians from various disciplines, managers, and to some extent patients. Both relied on well-connected vertically integrating cores, comprising individuals with credibility, authority, and strong backing from reputable institutions. Both sought to build a sense of community through, for example, meetings and virtual get-togethers.

- **Building lateral ties:** one community was much more effective in building lateral ties *across* its members. In the other community, most interactions were mediated through the core team. While effective in the short term, this created vulnerabilities for the longer-term sustainability of the community, which remained highly dependent on the core team.
- **Achieving effective action:** the two communities diverged in their success in moving their members from good intentions towards effective action. One focused its efforts on externally set performance goals that had to be met, and using the community as a supportive vehicle for their achievement. In the second community, a more diffuse set of goals, reliant on teams' own priorities rather than a common shared ambition, made it more challenging to initiate change, and to drive it forward sustainably through measurement, comparison, and feedback.

The clinical community approach recognises the power of collaboration and professionally led improvement, but is also explicit that some judicious use of control-based devices – including, for example, data to hold units to account – can be a helpful or even necessary complement to the collaborative ethos.[43] The experience of managed clinical networks (described in Section 3.2), of course, illustrates the risks of going too far in this direction.

The clinical community approach has been adopted and extended in clinical settings. For example, at Johns Hopkins Medicine in the USA, clinical communities are used as a forum to bring together a multidisciplinary membership with a focus on a particular population, clinical area, or patient safety issue in member hospitals.[44] Some success in the use of the approach has been reported,[45] though so far no trials have been conducted.

## 4 Collaboration-Based Approaches in Action

An extensive literature has examined collaboration-based approaches to healthcare improvement. Here, we focus on two of the most widely discussed approaches: quality improvement collaboratives and communities of practice. Systematic reviews and other studies in this area make clear that the evidence base for all collaboration-based approaches remains equivocal. There is still limited understanding of exactly which components of these complex interventions are most associated with change, and how apparently causal mechanisms operate. There is, however, a growing literature on how these approaches can be optimised to maximise their chances of making an impact.

## 4.1 Do Quality Improvement Collaboratives Work?

Quality improvement collaboratives have received much research attention, to the extent that they are now among the most studied of all improvement approaches in healthcare. However, one major weakness in the evidence base (in common with many other improvement approaches) is the risk of publication bias – that is, the non-reporting of studies that failed to demonstrate statistically significant improvement. Almost by definition, publication bias is difficult to detect or quantify. A second challenge, given the resource intensity of collaboratives (including organising events, getting input from expert faculty, and arranging cover for clinical staff to lead improvement locally), is establishing cost-effectiveness. Third, like many improvement interventions (see, for example, the Elements on evaluation,[22] the IHI approach,[23] Lean and associated techniques for process improvement,[46] operational research approaches,[47] and workplace conditions[48]), quality improvement collaboratives have some of the features of 'black boxes':[49,50] complex interventions with many components, which are often not made clear, and whose role in triggering the mechanisms that result in intended (and unintended) change is often left under-theorised or unexamined. A further practical and methodological challenge is that exactly how such complex interventions work is likely to vary by context rather than being exactly the same in every setting (see the Element on evaluation[22]). These problems are compounded by poor reporting of the actual content of the collaboratives beyond their high-level focus and organisation, and of the degree to which the planned interventions were carried out as intended in practice (their fidelity). As Nadeem et al. note, the lack of description of ingredients, of what they are meant to achieve, and of what they actually achieve in practice is problematic for the evidence base for collaboratives.

> *As QICs [quality improvement collaboratives] continue to grow in popularity, this lack of detailed information makes it impossible to replicate successful QICs, to ensure that adaptations of QICs include key active ingredients, or to determine whether negative outcomes are related to the quality and fidelity of delivering this multicomponent improvement model or differential efficacy of QICs for different [evidence-based practices].[51]*

A recent (2018) systematic review of 64 studies of quality improvement collaboratives, predominantly focused on inpatient care topics,[52] illustrates some of the problems. The breadth of populations and intended outcomes – and of the forms of intervention that have been given the label 'collaborative' – made it challenging to synthesise the findings. Though the collaboratives overall 'reported significant improvements in targeted clinical processes and patient outcomes', the size of effects varied greatly between studies, reflecting both the varied ambitions of the collaboratives and the diversity of primary outcome measures used. Studies with high-quality (randomised) designs were less likely to report a positive outcome than studies with weaker designs, and the authors note risks of bias in several of the reported evaluations. Most of the studies included claimed to follow the template set out by the IHI's Breakthrough Series approach, but how this was translated into practice was rarely specified.[52]

## 4.2 How to Make Quality Improvement Collaboratives Work Better

While the literature continues to suffer from notable weaknesses, some evidence about the features of quality improvement collaboratives that appear to be associated with positive outcomes has nonetheless emerged.[25,26,53] One of the most celebrated success stories for collaboration-based approaches is the Michigan Keystone project, which sought to reduce infections associated with central line catheters in intensive care units (ICUs).[54] It brought together clinicians from 108 ICUs across the state and provided them with training, periodic conference calls, coaching, and biannual statewide meetings. A before-and-after study of the intervention reported substantial reductions in infection rates.[54] A separate, retrospective analysis sought to shed light on the reasons for its success, identifying key mechanisms that appeared to be critical (Box 6).[55] It was also a prototype for the clinical communities approach described in Section 3.4.

---

BOX 6 MECHANISMS THAT EXPLAIN THE SUCCESS OF THE MICHIGAN KEYSTONE PROJECT FOR REDUCING INFECTIONS ASSOCIATED WITH CENTRAL LINES IN ICUs

- Generating the will for ICUs to take part in the initiative.
- Creating a networked community.
- Challenging the received wisdom that bloodstream infections are an inevitable risk of catheterisation, and recasting them instead as a social problem that is amenable to intervention.
- Developing, sharing, testing, and refining various interventions that can be used at the sharp end of care, particularly interventions that precipitate change in social and interprofessional dynamics, such as goal-setting meetings and a checklist.
- Using data effectively so participating teams can see where their efforts are having an impact, and benchmark their improvements against others.

> • Selectively harnessing 'hard edges' – more coercive features that complement the intrinsic motivation of participants by making judicious use of external expectations and pressures for improvement. These might include, for example, asking units that fail to provide data to withdraw from the programme, or explicitly ranking units to make clear which ones are falling short of the standards expected.
>
> Adapted from Dixon-Woods et al.[55]

An intriguing postscript to the success of the Michigan Keystone project – and one that illustrates the work needed to get quality improvement collaboratives to work – was the rather different fate of a follow-up programme that sought to replicate its achievements in England. The Matching Michigan programme, modelled explicitly on the Michigan Keystone project, reported a disappointing outcome: it had no additional impact on infection rates over the reductions already in train.[56] A process evaluation found that many of the mechanisms that may have made the original collaborative a success in the USA were absent in England.[57] In particular, the programme lacked many of the features necessary for collaboration-based approaches to succeed, in part because it was run by a government body, in part because of a widespread perception of a wider punitive policy environment, and in part because no real networked community emerged. Participants tended to view the programme not as a clinically led, peer-owned collaborative, but as another top-down, centrally driven initiative. These findings suggest that both the context for collaboration-based approaches, and the sophistication with which their principles are put into practice, have critical consequences for their effectiveness.

For further insight into how to make a collaborative work, Øvretveit et al. provide a helpful, if somewhat dated, contribution.[26] They identify ten key challenges associated with collaboratives and offer advice on how best to overcome them (Box 7). Hulscher et al. also offer practical, evidence-informed advice on how best to make collaboratives work.[25]

## 4.3 Do Communities of Practice Work?

Because communities of practice are a rather looser intervention than quality improvement collaboratives, the challenge of producing an integrated, coherent, definitive evidence base about whether they work is even harder. Consistent with their focus on the sharing of knowledge to inform professional practice as an end in itself, their objectives are often diffuse, and only indirectly related to

---

Box 7 How to get quality improvement collaboratives to work

- Choose a sufficiently specific subject, one that is strategically important to participating organisations, and one where sufficient evidence-based interventions are available as a starting point for the collaborative's work.
- Ensure that teams are properly selected and prepared for the collaborative, so they know what their objective is and they have the capacity to benefit from participation. Internal team dynamics can be crucial to each team's ability to contribute to and benefit from the collaborative.
- Dedicate sufficient time in collaborative meetings 'to facilitating learning by practice and to allowing teams to discuss how to apply ideas in the team's home setting'. Ensuring participating teams have the opportunity for two-way dialogue is more important than trying to compress 'too many didactic presentations into the meetings'.
- Motivate and empower participating teams by enlisting credible experts, providing good evidence, highlighting the human cost of suboptimal practices, and offering practical examples of how other teams have translated principles of high-quality care into practice in real-life settings.
- Ensure that teams have measurable and achievable targets for their work, including a balance between challenge and feasibility. Include mechanisms for feedback to the collaborative.
- Plan for sustaining improvements beyond the course of the collaborative, which may mean considering aspects of care that are not within the immediate control of participating teams, and spreading learning to other units and organisations that did not participate.

Adapted from Øvretveit et al.[26]

---

care outcomes; they may even defy measurement. Consequently, systematic reviews of the approach[58,59] have focused more on the question of what communities of practice look like and how they have been operationalised in the healthcare context, rather than on the evidence for their effectiveness.

In their systematic review of communities of practice in the business and healthcare sectors, Li et al.[58] found that those convening and studying communities of practice mostly took Wenger et al.'s definition as their starting point (i.e. 'groups of people who share a concern, a set of problems, or a passion about a topic, and who deepen their knowledge and expertise in this area by interacting on an ongoing basis'[38]). In practice, however, they found that the form taken by the communities varied substantially, often deviating from the original principles in significant ways. Key characteristics that might be seen as prerequisites for calling a group a community of practice – 'social interaction among members, knowledge sharing, knowledge creation, and identity building' – were 'not consistently present in all [communities of practice]'.[58] The authors were unable to find any credible evidence for the effectiveness (or not) of communities of practice.

A subsequent review, by Ranmuthugala et al.,[59] found a trend from descriptive towards evaluative literature over the two-decade period they covered. This review also noted that communities of practice tend to be one element of much wider change strategies, such that it was 'difficult to differentiate the impact of the [community of practice] component of the intervention from the rest'.[59] Three studies included in their review, including one randomised controlled trial, suggested that communities of practice were associated with improvements in certain outcomes. The trial[60] focused specifically on the uptake and implementation of an evidence-based standardised outcome measure for children's mental health, suggesting that, in the right circumstances, communities of practice can be useful in achieving improvement aims.

Nevertheless, there is a sense from this literature that the community of practice is best treated as what it is: an open-ended, largely self-organising process led by members, who are working towards ends that they define and that are not fixed. This is quite different from an intervention in the narrower sense of the term, which is driven by specified objectives that relate to improvements in the process or outcomes of healthcare. Yet there is also a sense, in healthcare and elsewhere, that the idea of the community of practice is increasingly seen as a 'knowledge-management intervention': a key part of an organisation's infrastructure that can help to aid the diffusion of information across units, professional groupings, and geographical boundaries, but which diverges even further from the idea of self-organisation and self-defined objectives.[61]

## 5 Critiques of Collaboration-Based Approaches

Collaboration-based approaches are widespread but have been subject to critique. One set of challenges is quite practical in character. It is easy to underestimate the level of operational, administrative, and infrastructural support necessary to achieve high-quality coordination of a collaborative effort, and the costs associated with collaborative interorganisational relationships may be significant but hard to resource.[62]

A perhaps even greater problem is that these approaches are based on the fundamental assumption that those involved in them take their obligations seriously, and will cooperate in good faith to achieve the goals of the endeavour. But the peer-based networks on which collaborations are based often have limited means of correcting those who fail to live up to these expectations. Ostrom's classic analysis[63] points towards the tensions between individual and collective interest in any situation where there is a 'commons' or shared resource (such as a collaborative, community of practice, or other network). Some form of oversight may therefore be a (regrettable) necessity, regardless of the arrangement for delivering or improving healthcare. But it can be difficult to achieve without reproducing the very hierarchical structures that collaboration-based approaches seek to bypass.

Exactly these challenges surfaced in a quality improvement collaborative in 2008–09, modelled explicitly on the Breakthrough Series approach. It aimed to improve the quality of stroke care in north-west England, as measured by key indicators in the English National Sentinel Audit of Stroke. A cluster-randomised controlled trial suggested that the collaborative was associated with modest improvements in relation to some of the process measures (compared with an ongoing positive trend occurring independently of the intervention, and possibly a contamination effect, which saw smaller improvements in the control hospitals too).[64] An accompanying process evaluation found that participating units contributed with varying degrees of enthusiasm to the collaborative, and identified factors that could stifle engagement and hinder progress.[65] Notably, some of these were issues of the kind suggested by social scientific theory such as Ostrom's.[63] For example, Carter et al. identified the phenomenon of 'social loafing' (whereby people working together tended to exert less effort than when working individually), as well as 'collaborative inertia' (the challenge of initiating and coordinating action among a diffuse social group). They also found some evidence of a 'free-rider' effect, whereby 'self-interested actors, acting rationally, may substitute their own goals for those of the group, so that collaboration is undermined by the self-interests of individuals as they pursue competitive rather than collaborative advantage'.[65]

Developments of collaboration-based approaches to improvement, such as clinical communities (see Section 3.4), have sought to learn and apply these lessons. By making use of hard edges and enforcing social norms – for example, by insisting on high-quality measurement and a degree of accountability – these latter approaches seek to reduce the risk that an overly idealised notion of humans' cooperative instinct may produce collaborative failure. Nevertheless, the literature suggests that there will be limits to the extent to which collaborative forms can draw managerial pressures to their advantage, especially when the goals of collaboratives are low on the list of organisations' priorities.[66]

Further challenges arise when collaboration-based approaches are superimposed on more hierarchical or market-based systems.[62] The example of managed clinical networks (see Section 3.2) shows how supposedly collaborative networks can retreat from their initial ambition of facilitating the sharing of knowledge across staff and organisations, and become instead appropriated as a tool for hierarchical imposition and acquiescence to performance targets.[34]

Some weaknesses of collaboration-based approaches are specific to the approach chosen. For instance, the tendency of some forms of quality improvement collaborative to focus on and reward rapid change can result in a wearying and inappropriate 'sprint race'.[28] The episodic character of Breakthrough Series collaboratives, for example – existing only for a defined period while a problem is tackled – may risk inhibiting the development of the kinds of cooperative, network-based relationships that are most likely to produce enduring capability for improvement.[52,67] The short-term, intense focus on single issues may also divert focus from deeper, less tractable issues in improvement. Further, the available evidence suggests that the run charts favoured by Breakthrough Series collaboratives are not always of good quality,[68] and may not command the respect and credibility accorded to more robust registry-based initiatives. In this light, the enduring infrastructure of collaboratives, such as the Vermont Oxford Network and the Northern New England Cardiovascular Disease Study Group, may be a more useful model for long-lasting collaboration and sustainable change.

The community of practice approach is not without its challenges, either. Some argue that by thinking of communities of practice primarily as a solution to the challenge of organising and applying ephemeral, tacit knowledge, there is a risk of subordinating the concept to managerial interests. Rather than offering a means for professionals to hone their practice through interaction with their peers, the community of practice is at risk of becoming:

> ... *a tool for management to manage 'knowledge workers' and experts. ...* *The idea that a large organization should create pockets of collaboration to* *counteract its rationalizing, formalizing tendencies seems entirely* *sensible. ... The ambiguity of whether this is genuine empowerment or the* *management involvement introduces a new form of normative control may be* *the key to why so many [communities of practice] fail.*[61]

Even if communities of practice manage to evade managerial control, they face, like quality improvement collaboratives, challenges from a wider institutional field in which vertical command and lateral competition can marginalise the cooperative ethos.[61] Though they are intended to be more-or-less self-sustaining and self-organising, and to require less administrative overhead, the organisation of work – including short-term contracts, geographically diffuse arrangements, and unstable project teams – makes it increasingly difficult for communities to emerge, organically or otherwise.[69] Their costs are difficult to estimate, and it is difficult to frame them in the cold, hard terms of intended outcomes, measurable change, and cost-effectiveness, making it hard to build business cases for their support.

# 6 Conclusions

Collaboration-based approaches offer much promise and are sometimes seen as offering a way of combining the benefits of bottom-up and top-down improvement. But, notwithstanding the aspirational, cooperative principles on which they are founded, they are not a panacea. Despite decades of research, the evidence base for collaboration remains insecure and contingent, hindered by the difficulties of establishing effectiveness and determining costs. While frustrating, this is perhaps not surprising. By their nature, complex approaches like collaborations are likely to work in different ways in different circumstances, and the fate and impact of such interventions lies at least as much in the hands of those leading them – and their enthusiasm, skill, judgement, charisma, tenacity, and sheer hard work – as in the design of their originators.[55]

Despite the problems with the evidence base, important learning has emerged that will be valuable to those seeking to use a collaboration-based approach. Some of this learning involves providing the right impetus to help a collaboration to organise itself while avoiding undermining its ethos through excessive control. As we have discussed, some collaboration-based approaches arguably suffer because they rely too much on the commitment and goodwill of their members, but others perhaps risk stifling the benefits of cooperation by grafting managerial methods onto the collaboration. A would-be collaboration preoccupied with addressing narrow, managerially determined objectives may represent the worst of both worlds, by diminishing authority and clout over network members, and inhibiting opportunities for building trust, reciprocity, and space for innovation.

The evidence also suggests a need for precision in some things and flexibility in others. It is clearly important to identify the improvement objective, and to have some idea of how this might be achieved and how progress might be measured. It is much less clear that adherence to a particular template (e.g. the Breakthrough Series approach or any other) will secure improvement. There are also signs that excessive focus on achieving aims within a limited period may be counterproductive: it is challenging to normalise values and behaviours like trust and reciprocity quickly, and long-term sustainability may rest on the longevity of the membership and infrastructure of a collaboration. Recognition of the wider institutional context is key: external pressures may distract from, compete with, or distort the goals of the collaborative, and need to be anticipated from the outset. In other words, the network itself – not just the collaborative processes and behaviours that are built on it – should be a focus for consideration and investment. That can mean, for leaders, giving the latitude to deviate from organisational priorities so that members of a collaborative can find their own purpose, lest they be reduced to a rather clumsy and instrumental means of achieving top-down priorities or managing tacit knowledge.

The range of participants in a collaboration-based approach is also critical. For example, including administrative and managerial staff may be important not only in ensuring that the full range of relevant insights contributes to collective knowledge and action, but also in creating the right kinds of collective commitments and securing influence higher up in organisational hierarchies. It is also perhaps noteworthy that the involvement of patients and carers is documented in few of the published examples considered in this Element. As discussed in the Element on co-producing and co-designing,[1] the participatory turn in thinking on improvement emphasises the importance of patients' and carers' perspectives to formulating interventions that result in improvements that matter to them.

Finally, health-economic evidence for collaboration-based approaches remains weak. Their impacts in some circumstances[52] do not necessarily translate into cost-effectiveness. The cost of collaborative events and of organisers' and clinicians' time can be high. The opportunity cost – the alternative uses to which healthcare systems might put their efforts, and their potential benefit – should also be considered.

All in all, and perhaps to be expected given the heterogeneity of both the forms they have taken and the functions they have served, the message for practitioners considering collaboration-based approaches is to see them as neither utopia nor dystopia. If they are to have a chance of success, it is crucial to find the difficult balance between defining aims, processes, and measures, and providing the space, time, and latitude to allow them to flourish.

# 7 Further Reading

- IHI[24] – further details on the Breakthrough Series collaborative approach.
- Managed clinical networks
  - Cropper et al.[35] and Edwards[70] – an overview of the background to managed clinical networks.
  - Addicott et al.[36] – a critical overview of some of the challenges they faced.
- Wenger-Trayner and Wenger-Trayner[40] and Wenger and Snyder[41] – accessible overviews of the key ideas underlying communities of practice.
- Clinical communities
  - Aveling et al.[2] – the theory behind clinical communities.
  - Aveling et al.[71] and Frank et al.[45] – case studies of clinical communities in action.
  - The Health Foundation[72] – learning report on clinical communities, summarising an evaluation of the approach.
- Broader introductions to some of the theories and ideas that underlie collaboration-based approaches
  - Martin et al.[13] – an overview of the history of clinical professionalism and the origins of collaborative responses to hierarchy and market.
  - Powell,[4] Börzel,[8] and Exworthy et al.[73] – conceptual overviews of the distinction between (and overlaps across) markets, hierarchies, and networks.
- The Health Foundation[74] – a learning report on effective networks for improvement, describing the features of effective networks, including common purpose, cooperative structure, critical mass, collective intelligence, and community-building.

# Contributors

Graham Martin led drafting of the Element. Mary Dixon-Woods drafted some sections and critically revised drafts. Both authors have approved the final version.

## Conflicts of Interest

None. Some of the work cited in the Element has been previously published by the authors.

## Acknowledgements

We thank the peer reviewers for their insightful comments and recommendations to improve the Element. A list of peer reviewers is published at www.cambridge.org/IQ-peer-reviewers. We also thank Dr Fay Gilder for her helpful review of the final draft.

## Funding

This Element was funded by THIS Institute (The Healthcare Improvement Studies Institute, www.thisinstitute.cam.ac.uk). THIS Institute is strengthening the evidence base for improving the quality and safety of healthcare. THIS Institute is supported by a grant to the University of Cambridge from the Health Foundation – an independent charity committed to bringing about better health and healthcare for people in the UK.

## About the Authors

**Graham Martin** is Director of Research at THIS Institute, leading applied research programmes and contributing to the institute's strategy and development. His research interests are in the organisation and delivery of healthcare, and particularly the role of professionals, managers, and patients and the public in efforts at organisational change.

**Mary Dixon-Woods** is Director of THIS Institute and is the Health Foundation Professor of Healthcare Improvement Studies in the Department of Public Health and Primary Care at the University of Cambridge. Mary leads a programme of research focused on healthcare improvement, healthcare ethics, and methodological innovation in studying healthcare.

# Creative Commons Licence

# References

1. Robert G, Locock L, Williams O et al. Co-producing and co-designing. In: Dixon-Woods M, Brown K, Marjanovic S, et al., editors. *Elements of Improving Quality and Safety in Healthcare.* Cambridge: Cambridge University Press; 2022. https://doi.org/10.1017/9781009237024.

2. Aveling E-L, Martin GP, Armstrong N, Banerjee J, Dixon-Woods M. Quality improvement through clinical communities: eight lessons for practice. *J Health Organ Manage* 2012; 26: 158–74. https://doi.org/10.1108/14777261211230754.

3. Goodwin N, 6 P, Peck E, Freeman T, Posaner R. *Managing Across Diverse Networks of Care: Lessons from Other Sectors.* London: National Coordinating Centre for the Service Delivery and Organisation; 2004. www.birmingham.ac.uk/Documents/college-social-sciences/social-policy/HSMC/research/diverse-networks-2004.pdf (accessed 14 February 2019).

4. Powell WW. Neither market nor hierarchy: network forms of organisation. *Res Organ Behav* 1990; 12: 295–336. www.researchgate.net/publication/301840604_Neither_Market_Nor_Hierarchy_Network_Forms_of_Organization (accessed 4 June 2020).

5. Brown JS, Duguid P. Organizational learning and communities-of-practice: toward a unified view of working, learning, and innovation. *Organ Sci* 1991; 2: 40–57. https://doi.org/10.1287/orsc.2.1.40.

6. Greenhalgh T, Wieringa S. Is it time to drop the 'knowledge translation' metaphor? A critical literature review. *J R Soc Med* 2011; 104: 501–9. https://doi.org/10.1258/jrsm.2011.110285.

7. Jones C, Hesterly WS, Borgatti SP. A general theory of network governance: exchange conditions and social mechanisms. *Acad Manage Rev* 1997; 22: 911–45. https://doi.org/10.2307/259249.

8. Börzel TA. Networks: reified metaphor or governance panacea? *Publ Admin* 2011; 89: 49–63. https://doi.org/10.1111/j.1467-9299.2011.01916.x.

9. Swedberg R. *Principles of Economic Sociology.* Princeton, NJ: Princeton University Press; 2003. https://doi.org/10.2307/j.ctvcm4g75.

10. Freidson E. *Medical Work in America: Essays on Health Care.* New Haven, CT: Yale University Press; 1989.

11. Yeung K, Dixon-Woods M. Design-based regulation and patient safety: a regulatory studies perspective. *Soc Sci Med* 2010; 71: 502–9. https://doi.org/10.1016/j.socscimed.2010.04.017.

12. Parsons T. The professions and social structure. *Soc Forces* 1939; 17: 457–67. https://doi.org/10.2307/2570695.

13. Martin GP, Armstrong N, Aveling E-L, Herbert G, Dixon-Woods M. Professionalism redundant, reshaped, or reinvigorated? Realizing the 'third logic' in contemporary health care. *J Health Soc Behav* 2015; 56: 378–97. https://doi.org/10.1177/0022146515596353.

14. Bate P, Robert G, Bevan H. The next phase of healthcare improvement: what can we learn from social movements? *BMJ Qual Saf* 2004; 13: 62–6. https://doi.org/10.1136/qshc.2003.006965.

15. Plsek PE. Collaborating across organizational boundaries to improve the quality of care. *Am J Infect Control* 1997; 25: 85–95. https://doi.org/10.1016/s0196-6553(97)90033-x.

16. Schouten LMT, Hulscher MEJL, van Everdingen JJE, Huijsman R, Grol RPTM. Evidence for the impact of quality improvement collaboratives: systematic review. *BMJ* 2008; 336: 1491–4. https://doi.org/10.1136/bmj.39570.749884.BE.

17. Horbar JD, Rogowski J, Plsek PE, et al. Collaborative quality improvement for neonatal intensive care. *Pediatrics* 2001; 107: 14–22. https://doi.org/10.1542/peds.107.1.14.

18. Finks JF. Collaborative quality improvement. In: Dimick JB, Greenberg CC, editors. *Success in Academic Surgery: Health Services Research.* London: Springer; 2014: 133–50. https://doi.org/10.1007/978-1-4471-4718-3_12.

19. Share DA, Campbell DA, Birkmeyer N, et al. How a regional collaborative of hospitals and physicians in Michigan cut costs and improved the quality of care. *Health Aff* 2011; 30: 636–45. https://doi.org/10.1377/hlthaff.2010.0526.

20. Womble PR, Linsell SM, Gao Y, et al. A statewide intervention to reduce hospitalizations after prostate biopsy. *J Urol* 2015; 194: 403–9. https://doi.org/10.1016/j.juro.2015.03.126.

21. Horbar JD, Soll RF, Edwards WH. The Vermont Oxford Network: a community of practice. *Clin Perinatol* 2010; 37: 29–47. https://doi.org/10.1016/j.clp.2010.01.003.

22. Tarrant C, Armstrong A, Ling T, Dixon-Woods M. Evaluation. In: Dixon-Woods M, Brown K, Marjanovic S, et al., editors. *Elements of Improving Quality and Safety in Healthcare.* Cambridge: Cambridge University Press; forthcoming.

23. Boaden R, Furnival J, Sharp C. The Institute for Healthcare Improvement approach. In: Dixon-Woods M, Brown K, Marjanovic S, et al., editors. *Elements of Improving Quality and Safety in Healthcare.* Cambridge: Cambridge University Press; forthcoming.

24. Institute for Healthcare Improvement. *The Breakthrough Series: IHI's Collaborative Model for Achieving Breakthrough Improvement.* IHI Innovation Series white paper. Boston, MA: Institute for Healthcare Improvement; 2003. www.ihi.org/resources/Pages/IHIWhitePapers/TheBreakthroughSeriesIHIsCollaborativeModelforAchievingBreakthroughImprovement.aspx (accessed 28 February 2017).

25. Hulscher M, Schouten L, Grol R. *Collaboratives.* London: The Health Foundation; 2009. www.health.org.uk/publications/collaboratives (accessed 28 February 2017).

26. Øvretveit J, Bate P, Cleary P, et al. Quality collaboratives: lessons from research. *Qual Saf Health Care* 2002; 11: 345–51. https://doi.org/10.1136/qhc.11.4.345.

27. Ogrinc G, Davies L, Goodman D, et al. SQUIRE 2.0 (Standards for QUality Improvement Reporting Excellence): revised publication guidelines from a detailed consensus process. *BMJ Qual Saf* 2016; 25: 986–92. https://doi.org/10.1136/bmjqs-2015-004411.

28. McLeod H. A review of the evidence on organisational development in healthcare. In: Peck E, editor. *Organisational Development in Healthcare: Approaches, Innovations, Achievements.* London: CRC Press; 2004: 247–72.

29. Amess M, Walshe K, Shaw C, Coles J. *Evaluating Audit: The Audit Activities of the Medical Royal Colleges and Their Faculties in England.* London: CASPE Research; 1995.

30. Ivers N, Foy R. Audit, feedback, and behaviour change. In: Dixon-Woods M, Brown K, Marjanovic S, et al., editors. *Elements of Improving Quality and Safety in Healthcare.* Cambridge: Cambridge University Press; forthcoming.

31. Royal College of Anaesthetists. National Audit Projects (NAPs). www.rcoa.ac.uk/research/research-projects/national-audit-projects-naps (accessed 5 May 2020).

32. Newman J. *Modernising Governance: New Labour, Policy and Society.* London: Sage; 2001. https://doi.org/10.4135/9781446220511.

33. Martin GP, Currie G, Finn R. Leadership, service reform, and public-service networks: the case of cancer-genetics pilots in the English NHS. *J Publ Admin Res Theory* 2009; 19: 769–94. https://doi.org/10.1093/jopart/mun016.

34. Addicott R, McGivern G, Ferlie E. The distortion of a managerial technique? The case of clinical networks in UK health care. *Br J Manage* 2007; 18: 93–105. https://doi.org/10.1111/j.1467-8551.2006.00494.x.

35. Cropper S, Hopper A, Spencer SA. Managed clinical networks. *Arch Dis Child* 2002; 87: 1–4. https://doi.org/10.1136/adc.87.1.1.

36. Addicott R, McGivern G, Ferlie E. Networks, organizational learning and knowledge management: NHS cancer networks. *Publ Money Manag* 2006; 26: 87–94. https://doi.org/10.1111/j.1467-9302.2006.00506.x.

37. Lave J, Wenger EC. *Situated Learning: Legitimate Peripheral Participation.* Cambridge: Cambridge University Press; 1991. https://doi.org/10.1017/cbo9780511815355.

38. Wenger EC, McDermott R, Snyder WM. *Cultivating Communities of Practice.* Boston, MA: Harvard Business School Press; 2002.

39. Kilbride C, Perry L, Flatley M, Turner E, Meyer J. Developing theory and practice: creation of a community of practice through action research produced excellence in stroke care. *J Interprof Care* 2011; 25: 91–7. https://doi.org/10.3109/13561820.2010.483024.

40. Wenger-Trayner E, Wenger-Trayner B. *Communities of Practice: A Brief Introduction.* 2015. https://wenger-trayner.com/wp-content/uploads/2015/04/07-Brief-introduction-to-communities-of-practice.pdf (accessed 24 February 2017).

41. Wenger EC, Snyder WM. Communities of practice: the organizational frontier. *Harvard Bus Rev* 2000; 78: 139–45.

42. Toulany T, Shojania K. Measurement for improvement. In: Dixon-Woods M, Brown K, Marjanovic S, et al., editors. *Elements of Improving Quality and Safety in Healthcare.* Cambridge: Cambridge University Press; forthcoming.

43. Aveling E-L, Martin G, Herbert G, Armstrong N. Optimising the community-based approach to healthcare improvement: comparative case studies of the clinical community model in practice. *Soc Sci Med* 2017; 173: 96–103. https://doi.org/10.1016/j.socscimed.2016.11.026.

44. Gould LJ, Wachter PA, Aboumatar H, et al. Clinical communities at Johns Hopkins Medicine: an emerging approach to quality improvement. *Jt Comm J Qual Patient Saf* 2015; 41: 387–95. https://doi.org/10.1016/s1553-7250(15)41050-5.

45. Frank SM, Thakkar RN, Podlasek SJ, et al. Implementing a health system-wide patient blood management program with a clinical community approach. *Anesthesiology* 2017; 127: 754–64. https://doi.org/10.1097/aln.0000000000001851.

46. Radnor Z, Williams S. Lean and associated techniques for process improvement. In: Dixon-Woods M, Brown K, Marjanovic S, et al., editors. *Elements of Improving Quality and Safety in Healthcare.* Cambridge: Cambridge University Press; forthcoming.

47. Utley M, Crowe S, Pagel C. Operational research approaches. In: Dixon-Woods M, Brown K, Marjanovic S, et al., editors. *Elements of Improving Quality and Safety in Healthcare*. Cambridge: Cambridge University Press; 2022. https://doi.org/10.1017/9781009236980.

48. Maben J, Ball J, Edmondson AC. Workplace conditions. In: Dixon-Woods M, Brown K, Marjanovic S, et al., editors. *Elements of Improving Quality and Safety in Healthcare*. Cambridge: Cambridge University Press; forthcoming.

49. Wilson T, Berwick DM, Cleary PD. What do collaborative improvement projects do? Experience from seven countries. *Jt Comm J Qual Saf* 2004; 30 (suppl): 25–33. https://doi.org/10.1016/s1549-3741(04)30106-1.

50. Shaw EK, Chase SM, Howard J, Nutting PA, Crabtree BF. More black box to explore: how quality improvement collaboratives shape practice change. *J Am Board Fam Med* 2012; 25: 149–57. https://doi.org/10.3122/jabfm.2012.02.110090.

51. Nadeem E, Olin SS, Hill LC, Hoagwood KE, Horwitz SM. Understanding the components of quality improvement collaboratives: a systematic literature review. *Milbank Q* 2013; 91: 354–94. https://doi.org/10.1111/milq.12016.

52. Wells S, Tamir O, Gray J, et al. Are quality improvement collaboratives effective? A systematic review. *BMJ Qual Saf* 2018; 27: 226–40. https://doi.org/10.1136/bmjqs-2017-006926.

53. Kilo CM. A framework for collaborative improvement: lessons from the Institute for Healthcare Improvement's Breakthrough Series. *Qual Manage Healthc* 1998; 6: 1–12. https://doi.org/10.1097/00019514-199806040-00001.

54. Pronovost P, Needham D, Berenholtz S, et al. An intervention to decrease catheter-related bloodstream infections in the ICU. *N Engl J Med* 2006; 355: 2725–32. https://doi.org/10.1056/NEJMoa061115.

55. Dixon-Woods M, Bosk CL, Aveling EL, Goeschel CA, Pronovost PJ. Explaining Michigan: developing an ex post theory of a quality improvement program. *Milbank Q* 2011; 89: 167–205. https://doi.org/10.1111/j.1468-0009.2011.00625.x.

56. Bion J, Richardson A, Hibbert P, et al. 'Matching Michigan': a 2-year stepped interventional programme to minimise central venous catheter-blood stream infections in intensive care units in England. *BMJ Qual Saf* 2013; 22: 110–23. https://doi.org/10.1136/bmjqs-2012-001325.

57. Dixon-Woods M, Leslie M, Tarrant C, Bion J. Explaining Matching Michigan: an ethnographic study of a patient safety program. *Implement Sci* 2013; 8: 70. https://doi.org/10.1186/1748-5908-8-70.

58. Li LC, Grimshaw JM, Nielsen C, et al. Use of communities of practice in business and health care sectors: a systematic review. *Implement Sci* 2009; 4: 27. https://doi.org/10.1186/1748-5908-4-27.

59. Ranmuthugala G, Plumb JJ, Cunningham FC, et al. How and why are communities of practice established in the healthcare sector? A systematic review of the literature. *BMC Health Serv Res* 2011; 11: 273. https://doi.org/10.1186/1472-6963-11-273.

60. Barwick MA, Peters J, Boydell K. Getting to uptake: do communities of practice support the implementation of evidence-based practice? *J Can Acad Child Adolesc Psychiatry* 2009; 18: 16–29. www.ncbi.nlm.nih.gov /pmc/articles/PMC2651208 (accessed 13 February 2019).

61. Cox A. What are communities of practice? A comparative review of four seminal works. *J Inf Sci* 2005; 31: 527–40. https://doi.org/10.1177 /0165551505057016.

62. Kirkpatrick I. The worst of both worlds? Public services without markets or bureaucracy. *Publ Money Manag* 1999; 19: 7–14. https://doi.org/10.1111 /1467-9302.00183.

63. Ostrom E. *Governing the Commons: The Evolution of Institutions for Collective Action*. Cambridge: Cambridge University Press; 1990. https:// wtf.tw/ref/ostrom_1990.pdf (accessed 14 April 2019).

64. Power M, Tyrrell PJ, Rudd AG, et al. Did a quality improvement collaborative make stroke care better? A cluster randomized trial. *Implement Sci* 2014; 9: 40. https://doi.org/10.1186/1748-5908-9-40.

65. Carter P, Ozieranski P, McNicol S, Power M, Dixon-Woods M. How collaborative are quality improvement collaboratives: a qualitative study in stroke care. *Implement Sci* 2014; 9: 32. https://doi.org/10.1186/1748-5908-9-32.

66. Stephens TJ, Peden CJ, Pearse RM, et al. Improving care at scale: process evaluation of a multi-component quality improvement intervention to reduce mortality after emergency abdominal surgery (EPOCH trial). *Implement Sci* 2018; 13: 142. https://doi.org/10.1186/s13012-018-0823-9.

67. Bate SP, Robert G. Knowledge management and communities of practice in the private sector: lessons for modernizing the National Health Service in England and Wales. *Publ Admin* 2002; 80: 643–63. https://doi.org/10.1111 /1467-9299.00322.

68. Benn J, Burnett S, Parand A, et al. Studying large-scale programmes to improve patient safety in whole care systems: challenges for research. *Soc Sci Med* 2009; 69: 1767–76. https://doi.org/10.1016/j.socscimed.2009.09.051.

69. Roberts J. Limits to communities of practice. *J Manage Stud* 2006; 43: 623–39. https://doi.org/10.1111/j.1467-6486.2006.00618.x.

70. Edwards N. Clinical networks: advantages include flexibility, strength, speed, and focus on clinical issues. *BMJ* 2002; 324: 63. https://doi.org/10.1136/bmj.324.7329.63.

71. Aveling E-L, Martin G, García SJ, et al. Reciprocal peer review for quality improvement: an ethnographic case study of the Improving Lung Cancer Outcomes Project. *BMJ Qual Saf* 2012; 21: 1034–41. https://doi.org/10.1136/bmjqs-2012-000944.

72. The Health Foundation. *Using Clinical Communities to Improve Quality: Ten Lessons for Getting the Clinical Community Approach to Work in Practice.* London: The Health Foundation; 2013. www.health.org.uk/publications/using-clinical-communities-to-improve-quality (accessed 5 October 2017).

73. Exworthy M, Powell M, Mohan J. The NHS: quasi-market, quasi-hierarchy and quasi-network? *Publ Money Manag* 1999; 19: 15–22. https://doi.org/10.1111/1467-9302.00184.

74. The Health Foundation. *Effective Networks for Improvement: Developing and Managing Effective Networks to Support Quality Improvement in Healthcare.* London: The Health Foundation; 2014. www.health.org.uk/publications/effective-networks-for-improvement (accessed 4 June 2020).

Cambridge Elements ≡

# Improving Quality and Safety in Healthcare

### Editors-in-Chief
Mary Dixon-Woods
*THIS Institute (The Healthcare Improvement Studies Institute)*
Mary is Director of THIS Institute and is the Health Foundation Professor of Healthcare
Improvement Studies in the Department of Public Health and Primary Care at the University
of Cambridge. Mary leads a programme of research focused on healthcare improvement,
healthcare ethics, and methodological innovation in studying healthcare.

### Graham Martin
*THIS Institute (The Healthcare Improvement Studies Institute)*
Graham is Director of Research at THIS Institute, leading applied research programmes and
contributing to the institute's strategy and development. His research interests are in the
organisation and delivery of healthcare, and particularly the role of professionals,
managers, and patients and the public in efforts at organisational change.

### Executive Editor
Katrina Brown
*THIS Institute (The Healthcare Improvement Studies Institute)*
Katrina is Communications Manager at THIS Institute, providing editorial expertise to
maximise the impact of THIS Institute's research findings. She managed the project to
produce the series.

### Editorial Team
Sonja Marjanovic
*RAND Europe*
Sonja is Director of RAND Europe's healthcare innovation, industry, and policy research. Her
work provides decision-makers with evidence and insights to support innovation and
improvement in healthcare systems, and to support the translation of innovation into
societal benefits for healthcare services and population health.

### Tom Ling
*RAND Europe*
Tom is Head of Evaluation at RAND Europe and President of the European Evaluation
Society, leading evaluations and applied research focused on the key challenges facing
health services. His current health portfolio includes evaluations of the innovation
landscape, quality improvement, communities of practice, patient flow, and
service transformation.

### Ellen Perry
*THIS Institute (The Healthcare Improvement Studies Institute)*
Ellen supported the production of the series during 2020–21.

## About the Series

The past decade has seen enormous growth in both activity and research on improvement in healthcare. This series offers a comprehensive and authoritative set of overviews of the different improvement approaches available, exploring the thinking behind them, examining evidence for each approach, and identifying areas of debate.

Cambridge Elements ≡

# Improving Quality and Safety in Healthcare

## Elements in the Series

*Collaboration-Based Approaches*
Graham Martin and Mary Dixon-Woods

*Co-Producing and Co-Designing*
Glenn Robert, Louise Locock, Oli Williams, Jocelyn Cornwell, Sara Donetto, and
Joanna Goodrich

*The Positive Deviance Approach*
Ruth Baxter and Rebecca Lawton

A full series listing is available at: www.cambridge.org/IQ

Printed in the United States
by Baker & Taylor Publisher Services